OBESITY SUPPORT GROUP FAQs

BEFORE AND AFTER WEIGHT LOSS SURGERY

by

Muhammad Asad

ISBN- 978-1-7335068-6-1

Obesity is a chronic disease. Millions of people are affected worldwide. Obesity is a risk for the development of many other comorbid conditions. Advances in understanding and management of obesity are happening fast. The best results are expected with a multidisciplinary management approach. This book will be useful for patients seeking bariatric surgery options. Handpicked commonly asked questions from numerous support groups are included with short answers. This can improve understanding and help patients make more educated decisions about their surgical procedures. I hope this book will be a valuable addition to the existing resources on this subject.

Table of Contents

GENERAL QUESTIONS

What bariatric procedure is best for me?

There are several bariatric operations available. Sleeve gastrectomy is the most performed bariatric procedure in United States. Gastric bypass is the second most frequently selected procedure. Adjustable gastric band and duodenal switch are some of the other available options.

Adjustable gastric banding is the least invasive bariatric procedure. However, long-term studies have shown a significantly lower weight loss with this option compared to other bariatric procedures. This has led to a decrease in its popularity. Few centers offer it as a primary procedure.

Sleeve gastrectomy is relatively less invasive than gastric bypass. The operation removes about 80-85% of the stomach and does not require rerouting of the small intestine. Vitamin deficiencies are less common after this operation than gastric bypass. Even though short-term complications are similar to gastric bypass, long-term complications, including ulcers and bowel obstruction risk, are less common. Therefore, more patients are choosing this operation over gastric bypass. Sleeve gastrectomy can be converted to gastric bypass in the future if needed. An average person can expect to lose 30% of their weight after sleeve gastrectomy. A 300 lbs. person will be able to lose about 90 lbs. over 12-18 months after the operation.

Gastric bypass is more invasive than sleeve gastrectomy. The operation involves creating a small stomach pouch and rerouting about 3 feet of the small intestine. This operation leads to more weight loss (40% of total body weight) compared to sleeve gastrectomy and is more effective at resolving diabetes mellitus. It is also better than sleeve gastrectomy in patients with severe gastroesophageal reflux disease.

The duodenal switch and its several variants are currently performed at only a handful of bariatric surgery centers. Other options are intra-gastric balloons, V block and Aspiration Therapy. These procedures are FDA approved but less effective than the above-mentioned procedures and are not covered by any health insurance plans currently. Therefore, they are only available to patients who can pay out of packet for the procedure.

In general, one person may be suitable for more than one operation. So, the choice of operation depends on the patient's unique medical history and weight loss expectations. All bariatric procedures are effective at helping patients lose a significant amount of weight. Overall, the risk of serious complications is small in the hands of experienced surgeons in patients who are compliant with postoperative instructions and follow-up.

Finally, the choice of the best surgical procedure for an individual depends on many factors. A decision is best made when bariatric surgeons and patients are working together to determine the appropriate procedure based on the patient's medical background.

What is the best bariatric surgery operation available currently?

There is no single operation that can take the crown of being ideal. Every procedure has some pros and cons. Some of these are technically more demanding. Others are easier to perform. Some operations have more complications and associated risks. Currently, popular procedures are sleeve gastrectomy, Roux-en-Y gastric bypass, and duodenal switch operations. Sleeve gastrectomy is the most done operation in the United States. Gastric bypass stands in the second position. The gastric band was once popular, but now it is performed less often. FDA has approved gastric balloons in the recent past. The intragastric balloon is a temporary method for weight loss. The balloon stays in the stomach for a few months, and then must be removed.

Similarly, a gastric aspiration system has been introduced. This operation has not gained traction due to the need for the insertion of a tube in the stomach operatively. In this case, the patient drains stomach contents through the tube after meals.

I had multiple abdominal operations, including abdominal wall hernia repair with mesh. Can I still have bariatric surgery, and what are my options?

Depending on the type of previous operations, a decision can be made about the available bariatric options. In general, bariatric procedures like gastric bypass and duodenal switch, requiring handling of the small intestine, may pose more challenges. Multiple abdominal procedures and mesh placement can lead to excessive adhesions (scarring) between the bowel loops and abdominal wall. This increases the risk of nicking the bowel during the operation. If there are no additional contraindications, the sleeve gastrectomy procedure remains as a potential option for such patients. Chances of successful operation are high in experienced hands. In many cases well trained surgeons can still do the procedure laparoscopically, however, the chances of conversion to an open procedure become significant.

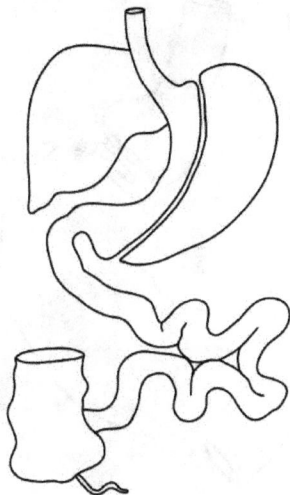

Figure 1 Sleeve gastrectomy

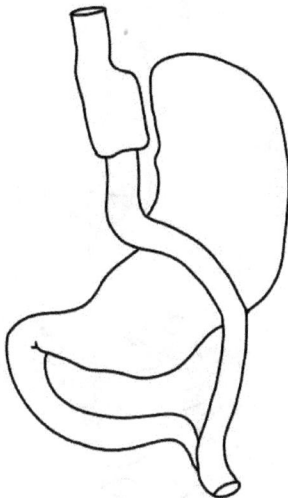

Figure 2 Roux-en-Y Gastric Bypass

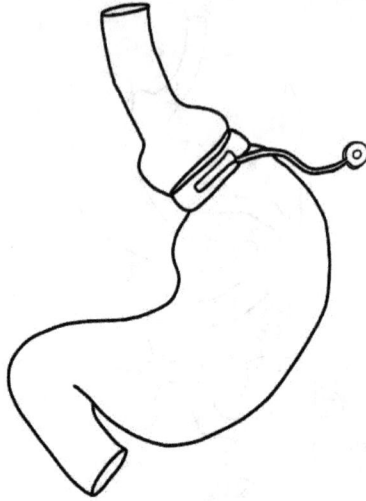

Figure 3 Gastric Adjustable Band

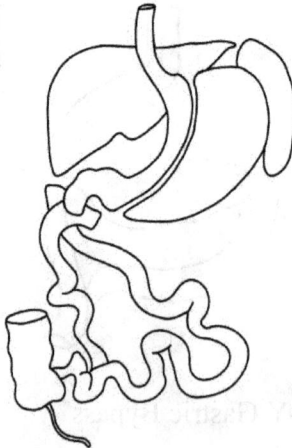

Figure 4 Duodenal Switch

QUESTIONS ABOUT OF BARIATRIC SURGERIES

I would like to know briefly about how common bariatric operations are performed?

Minimally invasive surgery has become the standard of care for bariatric surgical procedures. Most bariatric operations are preferably done with laparoscopic or robotic assistance.

Sleeve gastrectomy involves using a stapling device to shape the stomach to a small size. Gastric bypass involves creating a small stomach pouch from a bigger stomach using stapling equipment and rerouting about 3 feet of the small intestine. Duodenal switch operation is performed similarly. However, the stomach pouch is a little bigger, and a much longer part of the small intestine is rerouted or bypassed.

How does robotic surgery differ from traditional and laparoscopic surgery?

Robotic surgery is the next step in the evolution of laparoscopic surgery. The robotic system provides a high resolution 3-dimensional view of the operative field. Robotic instruments have multiple joints controlled by a computer interface that enables more precise handling of tissues and suturing of structures together. Robotic interface makes complex steps easier, and more precise. This advantage potentially translates into better results and fewer complications. Most bariatric operations can be performed with robotic assistance.

Does Sleeve Gastrectomy involve the placement of a sleeve on the stomach?

No sleeve is placed on the stomach. It is a misnomer. In this procedure, the stomach is trimmed with the help of a special stapling device by about 80 to 85%. The outcome is a small stomach. It can accommodate a small amount of food, thus helping weight loss. This operation also removes part of the stomach involved in producing a hunger hormone called Ghrelin. Patients are less hungry after surgery for many months, thus adding to weight loss.

What happens to the staples used in bariatric procedures and do I need to worry about any problems with staples?

Staples placed during bariatric surgery are made of a special alloy containing titanium. These staples are small and stay permanently in the body. In the short term, staple line breakage can happen in a small fraction of cases resulting in leaks. The body develops scar tissue around the staples during the process of healing. These staples do not cause problems in general, and no issues are expected at airports during the scanning of the body. Eventually, some staples can protrude in the lumen of bowel and may shed off. These staples are sometimes seen during endoscopy and can be removed if necessary.

Can I become allergic to staples?

Staples are not known to cause allergic reactions. However, there are situations when some staples may start protruding in the lumen of the stomach or intestine. By that time, tissues have already healed. So, removing them does not cause any serious problems or complications. If seen at the time of endoscopy, they can be removed easily in most situations with the help of special instruments through the endoscopes.

Do I need to take vitamins for the rest of my life after bariatric surgery?

Taking vitamins is essential after any bariatric surgical procedure. It is highly recommended to take the superior quality formulation of vitamins regularly. Simple over-the-counter vitamins may not be enough in many cases, thus resulting in various deficiencies. All bariatric patients are advised to have blood work periodically for different vitamin levels. Most vitamin deficiencies are preventable if the patient complies with postoperative instructions for vitamin supplementation.

Can I use vitamin patches on the skin, as I do not like most oral vitamin preparations?

The efficacy of vitamin patches has not been proven with a high level of evidence at present. Patients are strongly recommended to use high-quality vitamin preparations per the American Society of Metabolic and Bariatric Surgery recommendations. (www.asmbs.org)

QUESTIONS ABOUT GASTRIC BYPASS

What is a gastric bypass operation and how is it done?

Gastric bypass is one of the commonly done operations for weight loss. It was the most frequently performed procedure at one time but now it holds the second position. Gastric bypass is done with laparoscopic or robotic assistance. The surgeon creates a small gastric pouch the size of an egg. About 3 feet of the small intestine is rerouted or bypassed. The patient can eat only a small amount of food which fills up the small pouch very quickly. Food travels from the esophagus into the small stomach pouch and then bypasses about 3 feet of small intestine. The digestive juices do not mix with food till it has traveled through the rerouted segment of bowel. This adds to the malabsorptive component adding to the weight loss and better control of diabetes. More recent research has shown that bypassing the small intestine also causes hormonal changes that suppress appetite and improve diabetes control.

What are long term complications of gastric bypass?

Most gastric bypass patients do very well in the long term. Some patients who are not compliant with vitamin supplementations may suffer from vitamin deficiencies. Patients who smoke and drink excessive alcoholic beverages are at risk of developing ulcers where the gastric pouch is connected to the small intestine. Ulcers can lead to abdominal pain, nausea, excessive weight loss, bleeding, or perforation. Later complications may require blood transfusions, endoscopic procedures, or emergency surgery. Other rare complications include dumping syndrome and hypoglycemia. Weight gain is seen in a small percentage of cases who do not comply with postop diet and long-term follow-up. Many studies have shown that long-term follow-up with a bariatric program reduces the risk of serious complications and improves long-term weight loss and weight maintenance.

QUESTIONS ABOUT SLEEVE GASTRECTOMY

What is a sleeve gastrectomy procedure?

Sleeve gastrectomy is one of the most done operations in bariatric practices across the United States. The surgeon removes 80-85% of the stomach. This operation is done with laparoscopic or robotic assistance. Patients have short postoperative stays in the hospital, which is usually a couple of nights or less. Patients initially stay on a liquid diet and gradually advance to a regular diet over the next few weeks. On average, patients lose 30% of their weight after sleeve gastrectomy. The risk of serious complications is incredibly low in the hands of experienced surgeons. Early post-op complications include bleeding (1-2%), leakage from staple line (1-2%) and blood clots or DVT (deep venous thrombosis 1-2%). Long-term complications include development of gastroesophageal reflux disease. This procedure is less invasive than gastric bypass. Weight loss is slightly less with sleeve gastrectomy than gastric bypass (30% vs 40% of total weight). Vitamin deficiencies are less common as well. Patients are still recommended to take high-quality vitamins in appropriate doses.

I have severe gastroesophageal reflux disease (GERD). Can I still get a sleeve gastrectomy procedure?

Patients with severe gastroesophageal reflux disease may not be suitable for sleeve gastrectomy unless the reason for gastroesophageal reflux disease is known and treatable. People struggling with weight issues also commonly have hiatus hernias. If hiatus hernia is fixed while doing sleeve gastrectomy, the incidence of GERD may be reduced. A small number of patients have motility disorders of the esophagus and stomach. Their symptoms may mimic gastroesophageal

16

reflux disease. Your bariatric surgeon may request necessary investigations to check for these disorders before your sleeve gastrectomy procedure. In any such case, appropriate counseling can be done for eligibility for sleeve gastrectomy on a case-by-case basis.

Hiatus hernia is a condition where the stomach tends to protrude into the chest by varying degree due to a large opening between the abdomen and chest. This makes stomach contents, especially acid to, spill back into the esophagus, causing GERD symptoms.

Is sleeve gastrectomy reversible?

Sleeve gastrectomy is not a reversible operation. A small stomach is created with a special stapling device from the main stomach. A special technique removes the redundant part of the stomach from the body. The operation cannot be reversed; however, it can be revised to another type like Roux-en-Y gastric bypass or duodenal switch if needed.

Will I be able to eat everything after the sleeve gastrectomy?

After sleeve gastrectomy, the person can eat everything that anyone with a normal stomach can eat. Liquids are generally started on the same day as surgery. Food is gradually advanced to normal diet in 6 weeks with phases of liquids, semisolid (pureed) diets in the transition period. Portion size becomes less. The person feels full after a small amount of food. Hunger feelings are less as a portion of the stomach producing hunger hormone is removed during sleeve gastrectomy operation. It is an observation that food tolerance may change after bariatric surgery. Sleeve gastrectomy is no exception to it. Preferences for certain types of meats and bread may alter. Learning how to eat slowly is essential. Eating fast can bring discomfort immediately.

QUESTIONS ABOUT GASTRIC BAND

What is a gastric band operation?

The idea behind the gastric band is to place a silicon ring on the top of the stomach. The ring incorporates a balloon that can be inflated with appropriate fluid. This fluid is injected with a special needle to an access port through the skin to tighten the ring. The tightness of the ring part of the band limits the amount of food one can eat at one time. Band tightness can be adjusted as needed. This operation is usually done with laparoscopic assistance. Gastric band operation was popular in the past, but in the last several years, its popularity has diminished significantly for several reasons.

Why did gastric band operation become less popular?

Gastric band operation is considered as a high-maintenance option. It may require frequent visits to the bariatric office for adjustments. This costs money and time. Having injections at the access port site becomes painful sometimes. There may be a need for x-rays or endoscopy periodically to check the band integrity. The average weight loss is about 50 lbs. It requires serious lifestyle changes to make meaningful weight loss. High reoperation rate is reported in the literature. It may approach up to 50 out of 100 patients needing revision of some sort in 7 years. The band can erode into the stomach leading to infection. The slipped band can cause a blockage with constant vomiting. It may require emergency intervention. Chronic heartburn symptoms can develop due to reflux or motility problems in the esophagus. Poor weight loss is another concern. Some band access ports flip due to lose attachment to muscles. This may make access to the port difficult. X-rays may be needed in such cases for access to band adjustments.

QUESTIONS ABOUT DUODENAL SWITCH

What is a duodenal switch operation?

Duodenal switch is an effective bariatric operation. It is known to cause the highest weight loss. It is also highly effective for diabetes. In this operation, the surgeon cuts the duodenum with the help of a special stapling device. The small intestine is measured carefully, and an anastomosis is created at this level, and additional anastomosis is created at the level of divided duodenum. This operation can cause nutritional, vitamin, and trace element deficiencies. Fat-soluble vitamins are significantly affected by this operation.

In recent years, modification of the procedure is becoming popular. It is called single anastomosis duodenal switch. It is technically easier to perform with potentially fewer complications. It is also associated with fewer nutritional deficiencies. This procedure is recently recognized by the American Society of Bariatric and Metabolic Surgery as an accepted bariatric option. This kind of surgery is presently offered in a limited number of centers.

QUESTIONS ABOUT GASTRIC BALLOONS

What is a gastric balloon and how does it work?

Gastric balloons have been introduced in the USA in the recent past. This is a temporary method of weight loss. These are made up of silicon or similar materials. These are placed in the stomach. Most versions require the use of an endoscope. The balloon is filled to a specified level. This gives fullness in the stomach. It helps improve satiety and reduce food intake. This helps in weight loss. The gastric balloon stays for a few months, and later it must be removed. At present most insurances do not cover this procedure. Weight loss is mild to modest with this type of intervention.

CHOOSING THE RIGHT OPERATION

Which operation should I choose?

Choosing the type of operation for own self is a daunting task for many patients. One person may be suitable for more than one kind of operation. The decision can also depend on the types of medical problems present. A patient with a lot of gastroesophageal reflux or heartburn symptoms may not be a suitable candidate for sleeve gastrectomy. On the other hand, the presence of diabetes may make the decisive shift towards gastric bypass or duodenal switch operations. Anyone taking non-steroidal pain medications or aspirin may be at risk for developing gastric ulcers if they have a gastric bypass operation. They may be more suitable for duodenal switch operation. This operation is not susceptible to developing the kind of ulcers that gastric bypass patients may have.

The decision to select the operation type also depends on whether the patient had a bariatric procedure done in the past. Anyone with a history of gastric band can be considered for removal of the gastric adjustable band and conversion to either sleeve gastrectomy, gastric bypass, or duodenal switch. In some cases, band removal is done as a first step. A few months later, conversion to a different procedure is carried out in the next step. Similarly, anyone who has had sleeve gastrectomy in the past may need to be converted to a gastric bypass or duodenal switch operation for more weight loss. Anyone who has had a past gastric bypass or duodenal switch operation has only limited options for revisional procedures. Gastric bypass patients who have gained weight because of the technical factors related to the gastric pouch or its opening being stretched may be suitable for a revision. In recent years, a technique has been introduced where the surgeon can go through the mouth with the help of an endoscope and repair the gastric pouch and its opening with the help of sutures.

Some other older variations of gastric operations are not done presently. One of these operations includes vertical banded gastroplasty. This operation can be converted into a gastric bypass or sleeve gastrectomy procedure.

Patients are encouraged to have detailed discussions with their providers about the revision options.

HAIR LOSS QUESTIONS?

Which operation should I choose to have less hair loss?

Hair loss after bariatric surgery is a question that comes to many minds. Women are especially genuinely concerned about and have a great fear of losing their hair. Rapid weight loss after bariatric surgery is commonly associated with this issue. Gastric bypass, sleeve gastrectomy, duodenal switch, and other procedures which cause rapid weight loss are known to cause hair loss to varying degrees. It is hard to predict who will get more hair loss. Hair loss is seen in the first year after weight loss surgery. As weight gets stabilized, hair loss becomes less so. Most patients will see regrowth of hair.

What are my options to prevent hair loss and help them regrow?

In most people, hair regrow over time. It is a general recommendation that patients should improve their protein intake. Biotin use may be helpful. Sometimes, dermatology consultation may be needed to look at other specific and specialized therapies to help grow hair.

QUESTIONS ABOUT LIQUID DIET

How many days of liquid diet do I need to do?

The duration of liquid diet depends on the weight of the patient. BMI value, calculated from the patient's weight and height, is used for this decision. It varies from anywhere from 6 to 12 days. These recommendations are based on general guidelines. High-level evidence is lacking to prove long-term validity and outcomes of any such regimens. In general, patients with higher BMI (commonly more than 45) are required to do longer duration of low-calorie liquid diets. Different bariatric programs have crafted regimens according to their preferences. Patients should check with their program about the duration of the liquid diet needed. People are generally required to take four protein meal replacement shakes of approximately 160 to 200 calories each as their meals. It should contain anywhere from 25 to 30 grams of protein in each serving. Patients are required to take multivitamins and drink enough water. Sometimes they are recommended to take some broth preparation additionally to replace electrolytes. The primary purpose of doing a liquid diet is to shrink liver size. Experience shows that most patients tolerate liquid diets well. The state of ketosis, produced shortly after the start of these diets, makes people anorexic and not very hungry. In the state of ketosis is when the body starts burning fat stores. Special chemicals called ketone bodies are produced, which can be detected in urine and blood. Ketone bodies may also produce some smell in the breath.

People on diuretics (water pills) or taking diabetic medications should be careful while doing liquid diets for many reasons. Electrolytes and blood sugar need to be watched. Great caution is required with the use of any water pills during liquid diets, as severe dehydration and serious electrolyte problems can occur.

QUESTIONS ABOUT MEDICATIONS

What medications should I continue when doing a liquid diet before surgery?

It is essential to understand medications that are ok to take on days before surgery. Significant concerns are about blood thinners, diabetic medications, water pills, and some blood pressure medications. Additionally, one must pay attention to aspirin and similar class of drugs. Blood thinners constitute another category that needs attention ahead of time.

Practices and protocols vary from one program to the other. People are asked to stop metformin once they start liquid diets. Additionally, those using insulin are usually required to adjust the dose. This may also vary with your blood sugar control in previous days. Most programs work closely with family physicians and endocrinologists to help patients with complex problems to walk through the process. This is necessary to avoid hypoglycemia while on a liquid diet.

Ace inhibitors (examples include lisinopril and captopril) should be avoided while on the liquid diet. Some studies have shown adverse effects on renal functions while taking above-said medications along with a liquid diet.

Aspirin and blood thinners should be stopped appropriately before surgery. The former should be stopped about 7 days before the procedure. Other blood thinners should be dealt with their kind and necessity to use continuously. Sometimes a high-risk patient may need bridging with some short-acting injectable blood thinner medications. Patients are advised to check with their surgeon before taking any action.

QUESTIONS ABOUT ACTIVITY BEFORE AND AFTER SURGERY

What kind of Activity is permitted before and after surgery?

Any activity is welcomed. Jogging, running, treadmill, elliptical, or walking should be maintained pre-surgery. This helps in pre-conditioning the body. This makes it easier for the patients to endure operative and anesthesia stresses. Patients in most programs are provided with breathing exercise tools during anesthesia assessment visits. This allows them to get used to these instruments.

Patients are encouraged to get out of bed after surgery once they wake up from anesthesia. Frequent walking is encouraged. Light Activity should be continued in the hospital. It is vital to get out of bed and walk in the hallways frequently. Patients with disabilities get help from physical therapy staff to help them move. Restrictions are based on previous disabilities and type of surgery. It is expected that an average person should be able to resume activities without restrictions of weightlifting by approximately 6 weeks from the date of surgery. Most patients may be able to use stairs at home.

Anyone with symptoms of dizziness and lightheadedness should avoid climbing stairs to reduce fall risk.

What types of exercises are needed before and after bariatric surgery?

The type of exercise selection is a question that comes to mind while planning for bariatric surgery. In general, any exercise and physical activity is welcomed. There are indeed varying recommendations from different societies on this subject. These recommendations are mostly based on small studies. American Society for Metabolic and Bariatric Surgery recommends twenty minutes of daily exercise. It should be done three to four days a week before surgery. It may help reduce certain risks and improve fitness.

When should intimate activities be started?

In general, it is advised that when patients feel comfortable resuming their activities, they should do so with general precautions of not hurting the operative wounds with force and avoiding excessive bending, pushing, or pulling. For females, it is advised as a general guideline to prevent pregnancy for at least a year and a half after bariatric surgery. Precautions should be taken in this regard. Most practices advise patients to avoid taking birth control pills in the perioperative period to decrease the risks of venous clots.

ABOUT WEIGHTLIFTING AND WORKOUTS

How much weight can I lift after my bariatric surgery?

Patients are advised to avoid lifting more than 10 to 15 pounds for six weeks from surgery. Weightlifting limits and permissible activities may vary based on individual medical conditions and disabilities. Light Activity in the form of walking or jogging is permitted. Use of stairs is allowed in most cases. Resuming exercise should be gradual. Most patients should be able to resume activities without restrictions by six weeks from the surgery date.

QUESTIONS ABOUT POSTOPERATIVE CARE

What kind of care is needed for wounds or drains?

Laparoscopic surgery results in tiny operative wounds. External Skin stitching and stapling is done less often these days. Most surgeons like to close the skin with under-the-skin sutures that are not visible from the outside and do not need to be removed. Skin glues are getting popular, and these effectively seal the wounds, thus making showering possible very soon after surgery. Bathing or swimming pool activity should be deferred to a point at least when the wound healing has occurred to an adequate level. Wounds are mostly healed around three weeks after surgery. Many cases with revisional surgeries or some with emergency procedures need tubes or drains in the abdomen. If any patient has drains in place, the output of drains should be monitored and recorded appropriately. Patients are taught about the care of drains before discharge by hospital staff. Dressings should be changed as needed. Pets should be kept away from the tubes as incidences have happened where pets chewed the tubes. Accidentally pulling out the tubes is another concern. Tubes should be handled carefully. Anyone with a feeding or stomach tube should know about the blockage. If tubes are not flushed regularly, blockage is a possibility. In many cases, tubes can be opened with flushing. In some cases, tubes may need to be changed if attempts fail to unclog the tube. Most patients discharged with tubes in place receive nursing care from home health services. Accidental pull out of tube is a real risk with most drains. Patients should take utmost care and always keep the tubes, or their collecting reservoirs secure. There have been incidences where pets chewed tubes of critical nature.

It is vital to recognize wound infection. Symptoms of infection are in general pain, redness, and fever. There may be discharge of pus from the wounds or around the tubes. The fluid coming out from the tubes may look like pus. Redness of the wounds and around the tubes or any symptoms stated above should be reported promptly to your doctor.

QUESTIONS ABOUT SHOWERING AND DRIVING AFTER SURGERY

When can I take a shower and bath?

Showering is permitted within 24 to 48 hours (about 2 days) after surgery if wounds are adequately sealed with skin glue. Use of soap is allowed. Operative wounds should not be rubbed. Most patients feel fresh after showering. As mentioned earlier, wounds sealed with glue make it possible. Swimming or bathing should be done at 3 to 4 weeks to avoid wound contamination. Most patients have proper healing by the end of 3 weeks.

When can I start driving?

Driving can be resumed once patients feel comfortable and strong enough to make safe driving possible. In many cases, it is left to patients' judgment when they are comfortable driving. By the 2nd week most patients can drive. Driving should be avoided if one is taking narcotic medications and has symptoms of weakness, lightheadedness, or dizziness. Long journeys with a lack of moving legs should be avoided due to the risks of developing clots.

QUESTIONS ABOUT POSTOPERATIVE PAIN

What are my options for control of postoperative pain?

While in the hospital after surgery, it is not a significant issue for most cases. Some of the programs give pain pumps on the day of surgery. Patients can use the device pump for pain control at will. The amount of medication administered can be adjusted along with per dose in per hour limits. Oral medications for pain control are started on the first postoperative day. Most of the time, pain medications are in the form of liquids. Patients are very frequently advised to take some stool softeners as constipation is one of the side effects of narcotic pain medicines. Patients are discharged on liquid pain medications in most cases. Patients can take Tylenol for pain control.

A recent trend is to avoid narcotics. These medicines are known to cause significant nausea. Quite a few programs have started following recommendations and protocols suggested by the Bariatric society. This involves particular protocols to follow. Injecting numbing medications in the abdominal wall at the time of surgery is a helpful technique. It improves pain control with a reduction of opioid medication use. Depending on the protocol followed, patients may be required to keep a record of narcotic medications given to them and may need to submit the unused pills back to approved locations.

Many practices use elastic abdominal binders. Most patients report benefits from the use of these binders. use elastic abdominal binders. Most patients report benefit with the use of these binders.

QUESTIONS ABOUT POSTOPERATIVE NAUSEA

Why does postoperative nausea happen and how can it be minimized?

Postoperative nausea after bariatric procedures is common. The development of nausea is a multifactorial phenomenon. Pain at incision sites, effects of anesthetic agents, and narcotic pain medications are some of the contributing factors.

Several medications are prescribed to control nausea. Most surgeons like to use fewer narcotics and try to discontinue these medications as soon as possible.

At the time of discharge, patients are prescribed medications to control nausea. These could be in the form of tablets or liquids. There are preparations available where tablets can be placed under the tongue. These formulations are dissolvable and produce the desired effect of controlling nausea sooner. Some patients have reported benefits from strategies like aromatherapies. This modality is about the use of different fragrances to control nausea. Data is limited to prove the efficacy of this strategy.

QUESTIONS ABOUT A RETURN TO THE JOB AFTER SURGERY

I have a desk job when I can resume my duties.

Resuming duties after bariatric surgery is a common question by most patients. People are advised to plan for at least four4 weeks off from work. Many practices allow patients to go back to work earlier. Quite a few patients can return to work as early as ten days to 2 weeks or whenever they feel comfortable. Any release letters for the job will usually state weightlifting restrictions for 6 weeks after surgery.

I work for a factory and lift heavy loads. When can I join back?

Lifting weights of more than 15 to 20 pounds is restricted for six weeks. Drivers of heavy trucks, laborers, industrial workers, nurses, and nursing assistants are some examples of professions requiring heavy lifting weights.

QUESTIONS ABOUT MEDICATIONS

How will my medications change after surgery?

Many Patients are on multiple medications for several reasons. After bariatric surgery, a careful review of the list of drugs is made for every patient before discharge. Pain medications are prescribed to all post-operative patients. These are usually in the form of liquid formulations. Additionally, medications to control acid production or to protect the stomach from the effects of acid are needed. Frequently treatments for nausea and stool softeners are also prescribed.

Medications for blood pressure and diabetes require modification in most cases. For many patients, diuretics, which are water pills, are held for some time after surgery to avoid dehydration. Diabetic medications also need careful tailoring. An average patient requires a smaller dose of insulin than usual for reasons of less intake of food. It is also common to hold medications like metformin before surgery when patients are on the liquid diet plan.

Other common medications for depression, anxiety, or thyroid replacements are continued. If a patient is taking a lot of medicines spacing of medicines is helpful.

A specific challenge comes once the tablet size is big. Some formulations allow breaking the tablet into small pieces and taking it with a spoonful of apple sauce. On the other hand, some medications cannot be broken because of a specific type of formulation. In such cases, help from the pharmacy is obtained, and some alternative form of medicine, such as powder, liquid, or breakable tablet, may be selected. These issues are addressed before discharge from the hospital.

A special note is to be made for patients who get malabsorptive procedures like gastric bypass or duodenal switch-type surgeries. These procedures may alter the absorption of some medications requiring adjustments in doses, timings, or both. Commonly various services are involved in such decision-making. Pharmacists play a crucial role in such decision-making.

It is observed that some of the pharmacies in the peripheral towns do not carry uncommon formulations. It may be a convenient practice that patients get the fills of medications before they leave the hospital to avoid any hassle in finding the specific formulation locally from their pharmacy. Many hospitals have "meds to bed programs" which have been found helpful in getting appropriate medications at discharge.

QUESTIONS ABOUT WEIGHT LOSS EXPECTATIONS

How much weight loss is expected after my bariatric surgery?

Weight loss varies from person to person, and it differs for various bariatric procedures. Weight loss is rapid in the first few months and then slows down. In many cases, a stepladder pattern may be seen where weight may stall for some time. Weight loss starts again after a few days or weeks. Gastric bypass patients lose on average, 100 to 110 pounds of weight. Sleeve gastrectomy patients lose an average of 60 to 90 pounds of weight. Duodenal switch operation and its variations have a weight loss similar to or little more than gastric bypass. Adjustable gastric band patients lose an average of 50 to 60 pounds. Weight loss is also dependent on the metabolic rate of any patient. It is also highly dependent on activity level and dietary intake.

POOR OR SLOW WEIGHT LOSS AFTER SURGERY

Why do some patients have poor weight loss after bariatric surgery?

Less than 50% of excess weight loss is considered poor after bariatric procedures. However, any amount of weight loss adds some metabolic advantage. Weight loss is highly dependent on several factors. Two crucial variables are diet and Activity. Basal metabolic rate is an essential factor in the outcome. People consuming excessive amounts of high-caloric eatables, including chips, crackers, sweets, candies, chocolates, sweetened drinks, ice creams, peanut butter, and large amounts of cheese, may need to improve their eating habits to achieve their weight loss goals.

There could be some technical factors where some of the patients may have larger gastric pouch or pouch opening, stretched stomach after sleeve gastrectomy, or loose gastric adjustable band. Another situation is sometimes seen in gastric bypass patients where abnormal communications between the gastric pouch and the excluded stomach develop. This is called a gastric fistula. Many of these patients may develop recurrent ulcers in the stomach. A Fistula of this kind may cause loss of bypass effect due to abnormal channel. This may lead to poor weight loss. Similarly, some older surgeries like vertical banded gastroplasty procedures may have the opening of staples of the stomach leading to larger food intake and poor weight loss.

All cases of poor weight loss after bariatric surgery need careful review. Patients should check with their bariatric team for an assessment. In such cases, a multidisciplinary effort is needed to identify the exact reason and find a remedy if possible. Most patients of this category need some x-ray study to highlight the altered anatomy and endoscopy for assessment of the integrity of the stomach pouch.

NEED OF VITAMINS AFTER BARIATRIC SURGERY

What do I need to know about taking vitamins after Bariatric Surgery?

Patients need vitamins after bariatric procedures. The need is more in procedures involving malabsorptive components. Various formulations for bariatric patients are available. Bariatric-oriented vitamins contain higher amounts of different elements and other nutrient components. The American Society of bariatric and metabolic surgery has dietary guidelines for various vitamins on its website. Vitamins needed in bariatric patients include B1, B 12, folic acid, vitamin D, iron, and calcium. Trace elements like zinc and magnesium are required as well. Duodenal switch operations have specific requirements for fat-soluble vitamins, as absorption of this category of vitamins is altered with fat malabsorption. Fat-soluble vitamins include Vitamins A, D, E, and K.

A wide range of vitamin products is available. Patients must check with their bariatric surgery team to select the appropriate combination. It is also important to note that in the immediate post-operative period, many surgeons recommend chewable vitamins, which may be gummies or powder. After a couple of weeks, patients should be able to take pill or capsule formulations.

Most bariatric programs have protocols for checking vitamin and mineral levels intermittently. In the long term, once or twice a year, checking various vitamin levels and other components is essential to avoid deficiencies and clinical conditions.

I AM AFRAID OF COMPLICATIONS AFTER BARIATRIC SURGERY

What are common complications after various bariatric operations?

Like any other surgical operation, bariatric surgery is associated with some complications and risks. Overall, the incidence of complications is low. Some of the adverse events can be related to anesthesia or surgery itself. Some anesthesia-related complications include nausea, vomiting, sore throat, aspiration pneumonia, blood clots, and malignant hyperthermia syndrome. In pre-operative anesthesia visits, these complications are discussed in detail by the anesthesiology team with the patient. Bariatric surgery-related complications may include bleeding, various infections, formation of blood clots in major veins, dislodging and traveling into the lungs, small bowel obstruction, development of hernias, injury to abdominal organs, cardiac failure, and leaks from the staple lines. Some of the long-term complications include the result of various deficiencies. These may be related to vitamins and other nutrients. Patients may develop specific disorders associated with these respective deficiencies in such cases. Some patients may regain weight. A few other specific procedure-related complications may become concerning. Examples include slipping of the gastric adjustable band. Esophageal motility abnormalities, esophageal dilatation and aspirational pneumonia, band eroding into the stomach. Severe gastroesophageal reflux disease in cases of sleeve gastrectomy and adjustable gastric band operations.

41

PREGNANCY AFTER BARIATRIC SURGERY

When should I plan a pregnancy after my bariatric surgery?

Pregnancy should be avoided for a year and a half after weight loss surgery. This recommendation is based on consensus. Conceiving in the phase of rapid weight loss may affect the growth of the fetus. Females of childbearing age are requested to follow up with their family doctors or OBGYN physicians to select an appropriate method of contraception in the early phase after weight loss surgery. Patients planning for pregnancy should be aware of the unique needs for vitamins. They should also be mindful of the teratogenic effects of some high-dose vitamin preparations, including vitamin A. Prenatal vitamin regimen should be followed with intermittent checking of vitamin levels in patients conceiving after bariatric surgery.

REVISIONAL BARIATRIC SURGERIES

I had bariatric surgery in the past. I have regained weight. What are my surgical options?

Regaining weight after bariatric operations is not uncommon. All bariatric surgery candidates should never forget this fact. None of the bariatric surgery operations provide a cure for the problem of obesity. Bariatric surgery is a powerful tool. It must be used mindfully for the rest of your life to be successful. Those patients who have gained weight after bariatric surgery should have a thorough analysis to look at the causes of weight gain. A multidisciplinary approach is recommended for an appropriate review. Various eating disorders, emotional eating, and poor dietary habits should be addressed adequately. Patients should be assessed carefully about the operation which they already have. Any technical factors leading to weight gain need to be evaluated objectively. Various tests include gastroscopy, acid reflux determination, and anatomy review with x-ray studies. In general, a gastric band patient can be converted to a sleeve gastrectomy by removing the gastric band. Other options include conversion to a Roux-en-Y gastric bypass or a duodenal switch operation. Patients with sleeve gastrectomy with weight regain without risk factors to develop gastric ulcer can be converted to a Roux-en-Y gastric bypass configuration. A sleeve gastrectomy conversion to gastric bypass may be a reasonable option if reflux problem occurs. Primary weight loss surgeries have more weight loss in general. Revisional surgeries are associated with higher complications and more risks, including leaks. Comprehensive counseling is needed with the patients to make them understand the added risks and any potential benefits.

LOOSE SKIN ISSUES AFTER BARIATRIC SURGERY

Loose skin after bariatric surgery is a fear which everyone looking for weight loss surgery faces. People who lose more weight are likely to have more skin issues. Rapid weight loss may produce more loose skin. Younger patients are less likely to have this issue. Anyone beyond the early twenties may have less elastic recoil leading to more loose skin. Unfortunately, most insurance plans do not cover cosmetic procedures. Anyone with skin rashes, breakdowns, boils, fungal infections, inability to wear appropriate clothes, or to exercise may qualify for skin removal for medical reasons. Patients are encouraged to promptly report any skin issues to their family physicians and get these documented. Several patients report wearing elastic undergarments can make the appearance more acceptable. There are several commercial creams available claiming to reduce skinfolds and stria marks. The efficacy of these products has yet to be proven. Anyone opting for skin removal or any cosmetic procedure after weight loss must know that their weight should be stable for at least six months. Most plastic surgeons will consider cosmetic procedures a year and a half after bariatric surgery. For many people, the loose skin of the upper arms (bat arms) is more bothersome than the loose abdominal skin. Loose skin at the inner thighs can be troublesome in some other cases.

CAN I USE OVER THE COUNTER WEIGHT LOSS MEDICATIONS?

There are several products available over the counter with claims of causing weight loss. These products are sold in categories of dietary supplements and herbal products. Any such products are not endorsed by professional societies dealing with obesity. Some of the products can have harmful effects. FDA has approved only a handful of medications to help lose weight. Most of these drugs are prescription medications. Only one product is available over the counter, which is Xenical (ALI). Patients can discuss this issue with their healthcare providers dealing with weight loss.

WHAT IS ASPIRE ASSIST OPTION OF WEIGHT LOSS?

Aspire assist is a relatively new technique introduced in the recent past. The concept revolves around draining the stomach contents after eating. For this purpose, a tube is placed in the stomach. This requires a surgical procedure that involves implanting a specially designed draining tube system in the stomach. After a meal, the patient is expected to go to the bathroom to empty their stomach contents. Loss of calories results in weight loss. This technique has yet to receive significant traction due to the nature of the procedure and a cumbersome process that is unacceptable to many individuals. Insurance coverage is also a barrier for a select group of people for whom this may be an option.

SHOULD I DO FASTING/ INTERMITTENT FASTING?

Fasting and intermittent fasting imply consuming meals at certain times with significant intervals between the times' food is consumed. Fasting may allow the digestive system to recover and rejuvenate. It also improves self-control. Several studies have shown some health advantages with this technique. Intermittent fasting is done in different forms. It can be suitable for selecting patients. It is strongly suggested that patients should speak to their providers before starting any such practice. Patients with diabetes, heart issues, and renal problems and those on water pills have risks of some untoward effects if their oral intake is discontinued for extended periods. Numerous studies have shown a positive effect on body physiology and blood chemistry if fasting is performed in an appropriate way. Fasting is practiced in many religions in some form. American society of bariatric and metabolic surgery (ASMBS) has recently published its position statement on this issue, which can be looked at on the respective website. (https://asmbs.org/resources/asmbs-review-on-fasting-for-religious-purposes-after-surgery.

I AM AFRAID I WILL GAIN WEIGHT BACK AFTER BARIATRIC SURGERY.

It is a legitimate concern by some patients that they will gain back weight after bariatric surgery. Bariatric surgery is recognized as one of the most effective ways to lose weight and keep low. Data reveals that most of the patients will maintain their weight. It has been proven with numerous studies that maintaining a healthy lifestyle after bariatric surgery is associated with the maintenance of a healthy weight. Patients who have significant mobility problems due to joint or backache issues may see less weight loss. Some people indulge again in poor eating habits. Consumption of high-calorie foods and items with high carbohydrate content can lead to weight regain after losing. Frequent consumption of snacks, candies, sweetened beverages, and alcohol can make patients gain weight. It is strongly emphasized that adequate activity is maintained after bariatric surgery. Regular exercise with strength training helps build muscles and maintain a healthy weight.

A multidisciplinary team must carefully evaluate any patient gaining weight after weight loss surgery. They may need to see a dietitian, psychologist, or physical therapist. Starting weight loss medications at an appropriate time after bariatric surgery can help. A close follow-up with the bariatric practice remains essential in this regard.

WHEN CAN I TRAVEL AFTER BARIATRIC SURGERY?

The answer to this question can vary from patient to patient based on their medical conditions and how fast they recover. Long trips immediately after surgery should be avoided. Bariatric surgery brings significant changes in digestive anatomy and physiology. There are strict dietary requirements. Prolonged sitting in one posture can make abdominal wound sites painful. In addition, sitting for a long time without moving can increase the risk of clots in the lower extremities. It is encouraged if somebody travels soon after bariatric surgery, they should make frequent stops at rest areas or gas stations to have short walks. Activity requirements may differ for patients. It is highly recommended that patients should seek advice from their providers.

WHAT ARE GAS PAINS AFTER SURGERY?

Most bariatric surgical procedures are done laparoscopically under general anesthesia. Any procedure involving the stomach and surrounding areas, especially on the left side, can irritate the diaphragm and adjacent structures. Surgical dissection causes tissue trauma. There is a possibility of oozing blood. Laparoscopic procedures involve inflating the abdominal cavity with carbon dioxide gas. This gives space for the surgeon to work with the tissues and organs. After surgery, the abdominal cavity is deflated. Stretch caused by carbon dioxide inflation and operative trauma can make people feel pain in the left upper abdomen, shoulder, or back of the chest. Pain may be significant on the first postoperative day. It usually starts subsiding after that. With the implication of enhanced recovery programs and multimodal analgesia, most patients have very few such symptoms. General recommendations include frequent walking, breathing exercises, and reasonable pain control. There is no proven benefit with the use of medications containing simethicone.

SMOKING AND BARIATRIC SURGERY

There are strong recommendations for quitting smoking before bariatric surgery. Experience has shown that smoking leads to many ill effects on the body. There are numerous chemicals in the smoke. Patients who continue to smoke or restart smoking immediately after surgery are at increased risk of complications. Healing can be impaired with higher chances of leaks after bariatric procedures. Smokers can have various pulmonary-related complications. Lungs and air passages damaged with smoke are more prone to blockage due to secretions and injury to the lining with smoke. It may lead to lung collapse or the development of lung infection (pneumonia). Some insurances have mandated to quit smoking well ahead of surgery. They also force patients to join counseling sessions or wellness programs. Smoking after bariatric surgery can increase the risks of ulcers and heartburn.

WHEN CAN I START EXERCISING AFTER SURGERY?

Patients are strongly encouraged to start walking soon after surgery. Frequent walking and moving lower extremities improve circulation and thus may reduce clot-related complications. Once patients are discharged from home after surgery, they are encouraged to walk frequently. Light activity should continue. General limitations for weightlifting are in the range of 10 to 15 pounds for an average person. Too much pushing, pulling, and striking the surgery areas with force must be avoided. In most cases, normal activities can be resumed after six weeks from the date of surgery. Transition to full-scale unrestricted exercise needs to be gradual with incremental increase. Patients with severe mobility issues may have to opt for sitting exercises or need professional help from physical therapists for rehabilitation. For these reasons, some patients need to be placed in skilled nursing and rehabilitation facilities for at least a brief time. Patients must be careful and prevent falls while walking and exercising.

I AM SEEING STALL SOME MONTHS AFTER BARIATRIC SURGERY.

The weight loss curve can vary for different patients. Initial weight loss can be rapid. It slows down after a few months. Weight loss can be seen for up to a year or a little more afterward. Weight loss can vary with the type of bariatric procedure. In many patients, a step ladder pattern is seen. Some patients need continuous dietary and psychological counseling to counter excessive eating behaviors.

Patients with mobility issues related to musculoskeletal problems like arthritis may see slow or suboptimal weight loss.

Patients who lag in the weight loss curve must be carefully evaluated to determine the root cause. Some of these patients can be potential candidates for consideration for weight loss medicines. Several weight loss medications are now available, which are FDA approved. An inquiry with the insurance carrier can be made regarding the presence of coverage for specific medicines. There are a few commonly used off-label medications for weight loss. Patients are encouraged to discuss the issue of slow or inadequate weight loss with their bariatric team. In most cases, a multi-specialty team of qualified psychologists, nutritionists, and obesity physicians can help to achieve good outcomes.

CAN I USE WEIGHT LOSS MEDICINES BEFORE AND AFTER SURGERY?

Weight loss medications can be used in selected patients at any time during management. It could be before or after surgery. The data in this regard is growing. It has been observed that only some patients can lose significant weight during the preoperative preparation course. Some insurances do require losing a certain amount of weight before surgery. Most insurance companies do not see weight gain favorably during the preoperative phase. In some patients, consider the use of appetite suppressants. The choice of medication depends on many factors. Patient age, comorbidities, insurance coverage, and affordability are crucial in such decisions. In the postoperative phase, if the weight loss curve lags from the average, it becomes essential to identify the factors slowing down weight loss. A detailed dietary review should be done along with engagement of nutritional and counseling services. Weight loss medications may help some patients to maintain and improve their weight loss curve.

HOW MANY MONTHS TO WAIT BEFORE THE APPROVAL OF SURGERY?

A patient seeking bariatric surgery needs to undergo testing and optimization before the procedure can be performed. There are clearly defined pathways that are required to be followed. Various blood tests are done to check for multiple hormones and vitamin deficiencies. Blood biochemistry also reflects the status of the kidneys and liver and the presence of any anemia. There are educational requirements. Patients are engaged in various consultations and activities. Education about nutrition is one of the essential aspects. Patients are required to see a psychologist. Insurance carriers can impose specific requirements which involve monthly visits with their providers for counseling and education about weight loss and a healthy lifestyle. Such conditions can vary from different insurance carriers. Some insurances require up to 12 visits or more before surgery. On the other hand, some insurances do not require any specific number of visits before getting authorized for surgery. Patients are informed about such requirements at the beginning of the program. These requirements may also vary with each insurance carrier for their different plans offered. Some of the insurance will not require prolonged medically supervised diet visits for their members if their weight is remarkably high. The bariatric program coordinator checks such requirements and informs the patients at the beginning of the process. Patients can also check about any specific needs with their insurance carriers by calling their help/support line, which can be seen on the insurance card.

WHAT IS EXPECTED IN A PSYCHOLOGY VISIT?

Psychological clearance is one of the essential steps in the preparation process for bariatric surgery. Here the psychologist makes an independent evaluation of how suitable a patient is for bariatric surgery. A key part of the interview is about testing the necessary knowledge about the bariatric surgery procedure and knowledge about alternate options. It is expected that patients can express the basic details of various surgical procedures. For example, a sleeve gastrectomy involves shaping the stomach with a stapling device to create a new stomach size, like a banana or a sausage. About 85% of the stomach is removed. The patient will consume a small portion and is expected to be less hungry. A gastric bypass involves making a small stomach pouch of about one-ounce size and rerouting the small bowel to create a bypass of food from other parts of the stomach, duodenum, and part of the following small bowel. This operation cuts the portion size of food and causes malabsorption.

On the other hand, duodenal switch operation involves a similar component as sleeve gastrectomy and dividing the duodenum with the rerouting of the bowel contents to the later part of the intestine. A gastric adjustable band involves placing a silicon device on the top of the stomach. This device has a balloon-like structure that can be filled through an access port attached to the tubing and placed under the skin on one of the sides of the abdomen. Surgeon can inject fluid into the excess port to tighten the band. This procedure is done less commonly now due to various concerns about complications, durability, and less weight loss. It is also expected that patients may have brief knowledge about some of the other available alternate options, like gastric balloons. Patients are expected to be knowledgeable and able to express some complications which

56

can happen with bariatric procedures. They should be able to talk about complications like bleeding, infections, clots, leaks, and nutritional deficiencies. Psychologists also ask about the stressors and their social / family support. They also like to judge how strong the commitment towards a healthy lifestyle exists. They also inquire about previous attempts to lose weight and their outcome. Questions are asked about the use of alcohol dependence and any drug abuse. Psychologists do make comments about any mental disorders, especially anxiety, depression, bipolar disorder, and any suicidal ideation. A detailed review of any eating disorders is done. Common eating disorders include skipping meals, excessive snacking, binge eating, grazing, late night eating. Psychologists also comment about activity level, smoking, and use of recreational medicines.

Most psychology assessment failures happen due to a lack of adequate knowledge about the surgical process. Some patients fail to get clearance for surgery due to uncontrolled mental disorders. Those who cannot clear the psychology evaluation are provided additional education about the surgical process, nutritional needs, and potential complications. Depending on the condition, they may have further sessions with the psychologist.

WHY I SHOULD BE TESTED FOR SLEEP APNEA BEFORE SURGERY?

Sleep apnea is a clinical condition where an affected person has low oxygen levels during sleep. The patient cannot sleep well and wakes up with fatigue and tiredness. Daytime sleepiness can be another symptom in people who have obstructive sleep apnea. The healing of tissues is highly dependent on good oxygen levels. Strong recommendations exist regarding the need for testing for sleep apnea before bariatric surgery. The risk of poor healing and leak increases in patients with untreated sleep apnea. A sleep study is needed as part of the workup for sleep apnea. Nowadays the option of a home sleep study test is available. Those who are found to have sleep apnea on the screening test are subject to a formal sleep study, also called a titration study. It is done in a dedicated sleep center. Special machines are available to help generate pressure through the mask to keep the Airways open during sleep. Sleep apnea improves in more than 70% of people after weight loss surgery. Untreated sleep apnea has been implicated in several conditions, including fatigue, irritability, attention and behavior issues, cardiac arrhythmias, especially atrial fibrillation, pulmonary hypertension, coronary artery disease.

ADDRESSING CONSTIPATION IN PERIOPERATIVE PERIOD

Constipation remains a prominent issue in perioperative care during bariatric surgery. Worsening of Constipation can happen before surgery once a liquid diet is used. High-protein liquid diets do not contain fiber. Dehydration with less water intake can worsen the situation. Patients are encouraged to take stool softeners regularly. During and after surgery, narcotics used for pain control can contribute to this problem. These medications slow down bowel activity and may lead to the worsening of the condition. If constipation is not addressed adequately, hard stools can get backed up, creating a painful condition. This may require sometimes visiting the emergency room to have disimpaction. Most patients in the post-operative phase are advised to take stool softeners regularly. They need to stay well hydrated.

IS IT POSSIBLE TO STRETCH THE GASTRIC POUCH AND SLEEVE?

The size of the gastric sleeve or pouch does have implications. There is some correlation between weight loss and the size of the stomach reservoir. The expected size of the gastric pouch is around one ounce. The sleeve can hold anywhere from two to five ounces of food. Over time, some degree of stretching is expected in either of the bariatric surgical options. Any patient with poor weight loss or regain after bariatric surgery needs a comprehensive and multidisciplinary approach to identify the factors leading to weight gain. In many cases, poor eating habits are the main reason. Any patient suspected to have stretched gastric pouch or sleeve needs to be thoroughly evaluated for other technical reasons which can lead to weight gain. Commonly used tests to evaluate the pouch size include upper gastrointestinal endoscopic (gastroscopy) examination and special X-ray studies. The latter include contrast X-ray studies, including barium swallow and follow-through studies. Additionally, consultations with the nutritionist and psychologist are helpful.

IS GALLBLADDER REMOVAL NECESSARY WITH BARIATRIC SURGERY?

The gallbladder is an organ that is present under the liver. It stores bile. The gallbladder can develop gallstones. Risk is higher in people who are overweight. A normal gallbladder does not need to be removed at the time of the bariatric procedure. Most bariatric surgeons favor this option. In cases with documented stones or gallbladder dysfunction, performing gallbladder removal may be feasible at the time of the bariatric procedure. There has been a difference of opinions regarding this approach among bariatric surgeons. Difficulties can be due to high BMI (body mass index) and liver size. The risk of certain complications like bleeding, injuries, or bile leakage may increase. When signing the consent for the bariatric procedure, surgeons address this issue. Suppose a diseased gallbladder is removed at the time of bariatric surgery. In that case, it can avoid another surgical procedure and general anesthesia in the future. Many bariatric surgeons perform preoperative imaging studies to rule out gallbladder problems. This becomes more important if the patient has some gallbladder-related symptoms, such as pain or discomfort on the right side or upper abdomen. Ultrasound is a commonly done imaging study in this regard. It must be remembered that specific bariatric procedures like gastric bypass or duodenal switch operations change the anatomy of the digestive system. In such cases, direct access to the stomach or duodenum at the bile drainage duct opening may not be possible by the gastroenterologist. This can pose specific challenges. More complex procedures are needed to clear the bile duct stones in these cases. After Bariatric surgery, most patients lose a significant amount of weight by mobilizing various lipids from the fat stores. This may increase the chances of the development of gallstones by up to 30%. Medications like actigall may help reduce the chances of forming gallstones. It has been noted that compliance with this medication, in general, may not be high due to potential gastrointestinal side effects. The risk of developing gallstones may be increased in the first six months of surgery.

ISSUES OF CONSUMPTION OF ALCOHOL AFTER BARIATRIC SURGERY

Bariatric operations change the stomach's capacity and, depending on the type of operation, may also produce a malabsorption mechanism. There is a significant change in the dynamics of the flow of food contents. A normal stomach can dump a considerable amount of food. This is true for alcohol as well. Alcohol can reach the small bowel quickly in a person who has gastric bypass. It is absorbed into the blood and can affect the brain much earlier than in a person with a normal stomach. Risks of addiction can be higher in patients who have bariatric surgery, especially gastric bypass-type procedures.

Vitamin and nutritional deficiencies can be seen in patients who consume alcoholic beverages excessively. Thiamine deficiency can have several harmful effects. Patients can encounter nervous system or heart-related complications. Some patients can develop pancreatitis or fatty change in the liver. Alcoholic beverages can contain a sizable number of calories. Weight gain after weight loss surgery can occur if alcoholic beverages are consumed in larger amounts.

WEIGHT REGAIN AFTER SURGERY AND HOW TO AVOID IT?

Bariatric surgeries provide a great tool to help lose weight. However, these procedures do not offer a cure for the problem. Patients have a window of time that goes to approximately a year when they lose weight actively. Some patients cannot stay on track and opting for healthy lifestyle changes is hard. This group of patients is at risk of regaining weight. Uncontrolled depression, lack of rest, lack of sleep, poor meal planning, financial issues, and stresses related to family, relations, and jobs are important. Skipping meals with frequent grazing and consuming high-calorie food items, especially sweetened beverages, remains a significant risk of poor weight loss or regaining.

Some patients consume alcohol in excessive amounts. Significant weight regain can happen with any combination of the above factors.

Some medications tend to increase weight gain. These can be discussed at the pre-operative visits.

Lastly, lack of activity and exercise leads to deconditioning. Loss of muscle mass can decrease the basal metabolic rate making it hard to lose weight and the potential to regain it quickly.

It is highly recommended that patients follow closely with their bariatric surgery program after their procedures. Any patient lagging in the weight loss curve can be counseled, educated, and potentially placed on anti-obesity medications.

QUESTIONS ABOUT POOR WEIGHT LOSS

Any patient losing less weight after surgery needs a thorough evaluation by the bariatric treating team. Depending upon the type of bariatric surgery, a patient may lose a certain amount of weight. During post-operative surgery visits, this progress can be closely monitored. Generally, losing less than 50% of excess body weight is considered less than optimal. In most cases, weight loss can continue for up to a year. In the initial months, weight loss is rapid; however, as time passes the rate of weight loss becomes slow. It is common to see a step ladder pattern. Patients may experience plateaus for a variable period, ranging from a few days to weeks. This remains a concerning issue for most patients. Common factors include the consumption of high-caloric food items. Liquid calories in sweetened beverages remain a key factor in poor weight loss or regain after surgery. Snacking and grazing habits may come back. Another factor is lack of exercise and activity. Patients who are not mobile or less active have less than average weight loss, and their potential to gain weight remains high. In all such cases, appropriate counseling and referrals play a significant role. In select patients, appetite suppressants and weight loss medications may help. Various drugs are available. Patients should discuss with their providers about all such options. A multidisciplinary effort is needed for these patients. Such multidisciplinary teams include bariatric physicians, nurses, nutritionists, psychologists, and physical therapists. Most patients who keep up with the appointments and follow regularly can expect a good outcome.

HOW MUCH WEIGHT LOSS NEEDED BEFORE WEIGHT LOSS SURGERY?

Most programs require their patients to lose some weight before the bariatric procedure. Patients undergo various investigations, and it is mandatory to participate in educational activities about the expected surgical procedures and alternate choices. Patients are expected to lose at least some weight with this strategy before surgery. Current requirements of losing a certain amount of weight, as imposed by some insurance carriers, are not backed by large data-proven studies. It remains concerning if a patient seeking weight loss surgery starts gaining weight while in the program reflecting poor compliance. Any patient gaining weight or not able to lose some weight will require careful evaluation by the bariatric multidisciplinary team. Such patients need additional counseling and education. Sometimes surgery can get delayed for the same reasons. Dietary changes needed to lose weight include:

- Cutting down portion sizes

- Making the meals balanced

- Eating at appropriate times

- Avoiding grazing and consumption of high-caloric food items

Activity level remains a significant factor in weight loss and weight maintenance. Patients are always encouraged to increase walking in exercise. Unfortunately, some patients have limitations due to muscular-skeletal pains. Physical therapy, swing pool activities, and sitting exercises may help.

WHILE ON LIQUID DIET BEFORE SURGERY WHAT ELSE I CAN TAKE?

Most bariatric programs like their patients to be on a low-calorie and low-carb diet for some days before surgery. Especially patients with high BMI need to lose weight to make their surgery safer. High protein meal replacement shakes are used as the sole dietary resource. Several products are available. Protein meal replacement shakes generally have 200 or fewer calories and carry around 30 grams of protein. Patients can drink water or consume bouillon to replenish electrolytes. Consuming any other form of food or calories can compromise the expected results. The primary purpose is to shrink the liver size. Patients often talk about sugar-free jelly and popsicles. Ideally, all additional sources of calories in any form should be avoided. However, every effort must be made to keep hydration status fair. Although this practice of high protein meal replacement shakes for a variable time depending on the BMI is practiced by most programs. Still, there needs to be more high-quality data in support of such practices. The bariatric surgeon may decide not to have a liquid diet in selected patients. This is commonly seen in cases with low BMI or patients with abnormalities in the metabolic system. In cases with impaired cardiac or renal functions and people with diabetes, modifications may be needed in the liquid diet plan if prescribed.

The patient should check with their bariatric team for advice in this regard in their preoperative visits.

WHAT ITEMS SHOULD I BRING WHEN I COME FOR SURGERY?

Many hospitals provide a checklist for preoperative preparation and items to bring to the hospital.

The following are the everyday items which can make your stay more comfortable.

- Your CPAP machine (if you have sleep apnea and use the machine at home)
- Cell phone and tablet with the respective chargers.
- It is convenient if a long charging cable or an extension cord with multiple plugins is available.
- It is convenient to have your headphones. It will be a plus if you have noise-canceling headphones.
- Reading books.
- Reading glasses if you need one.
- Skin moisturizing cream/ lotion and ChapStick.
- In the summer season, a small portable battery-operated fan is helpful. Some hospitals provide this to their patients.
- A set of comfortable undergarments, pair of socks, and pajamas. A sizeable loose T-shirt is helpful to wear as you leave the hospital. It can accommodate an abdominal elastic binder if you get one. Slip-in shoes will help you wear them without bending.
- Toiletries Including mouthwash, toothpaste, toothbrush, body wash, dental floss, shampoo, and conditioner. Moisturizing lotion. A comb or hairbrush, slippers/flip flops, and any personal hygiene items.
- A blanket and pillow of your choice, although hospitals do provide blankets and pillows.

WHAT MEDICATIONS SHOULD I STOP BEFORE SURGERY?

This issue should be carefully sorted out before bariatric surgery in the preoperative visits. Patients can be on several medications. Some medications are required to be stopped. In general, blood thinners of any kind need to be stopped well ahead of time.

Commonly used anticoagulation medicines are aspirin, Plavix, Xarelto, Eliquis, and warfarin.

In diabetic patients, modification of antidiabetic medications is generally needed. Dose installation may need to be reduced. Some medicines may require discontinuation altogether. Patients are required to monitor their blood sugar closely in this phase.

Many bariatric surgeons would discontinue oral contraceptives ahead of surgery due to the risks of clots. Products containing estrogen may increase the risk of clots.

Patients on immune-modulating medications commonly used in autoimmune disorders need to be counseled carefully about discontinuing the drug. One of the common examples is methotrexate which is used in cases of rheumatoid arthritis.

The use of steroids can impair healing.

A careful medical reconciliation is made in the preoperative visits regarding the above-stated facts.

Patients are encouraged to check with their treating team if there is any confusion about continuing or discontinuing any medication.

WHAT CAN I TAKE ON THE MORNING OF DATY OF SURGERY

Enhanced recovery protocols practiced in most programs these days allow patients to take clear liquids up to a few hours before surgery. Liquids containing sugar are recommended by some anesthesia teams as it is beneficial in preventing insulin resistance. Non clear liquids like protein shakes should not be consumed prior to surgery as this will increase the risk of aspiration. This may cancel or delay your surgery as well.

WHY IT IS IMPORTANT TO MAINTAIN FOOD JOURNAL?

One of the significant factors in weight gain and the development of obesity is eating more than your body can burn. Food journaling is an effective strategy for documenting your intake. It allows you to do an audit with potential remedy measures. A food journal can be done on a simple notebook or piece of paper and maintained in a file. There are many apps available on smartphones. These can be downloaded from app stores by apple, google, and third parties.

It has been observed that patients who keep their record of caloric intake are likely to lose more weight.

DID NEW SHOTS MAKE SURGERY UNNECESSARY

A couple of injectable weight loss medicines are FDA approved and available now. These are effective in weight loss. Certainly, these are not replacing surgery. Average weight loss is expected to be 5 to 10%. Data has proved more and sustained weight loss with surgical options.

Best weight loss results are expected with multidisciplinary approaches. More and more bariatric surgery patients are opting for weight loss medications in their weight loss journeys. This could be in before or more often post-surgery phase.

www.ingramcontent.com/pod-product-compliance
Lightning Source LLC
Chambersburg PA
CBHW060519280326
41933CB00014B/3034